Get Moving,
Keep Moving

Real world lessons on fitness, happiness,
and healthy living

Dominic Lucibello

Published by Fitness Marketing Group, Sunrise Beach, MO.

Printed in the United States of America

ISBN: 9798443822648

This publication is designed to provide accurate and authoritative information with regard to the subject matter covered. It is sold with the understanding that the publisher is not engaged in rendering legal, accounting, or other professional advice. If legal advice or other expert assistance is required, the services of a competent professional should be sought.

First edition

For more information, contact:

Breakthrough
Fitness-
269 Aulin Avenue Suite 1011
Oviedo, FL 32765

1 (407) 542-5910

Visit us online at: www.breakthroughfitnessfl.com

TABLE OF CONTENTS

INTRODUCTION

Hi, I'm Coach Dom. My expertise lies in helping busy adults live a healthy, high-quality life. This involves the five tools of change- strength training, improving mindset, better nutrition, cardiovascular conditioning and R&R - recovery and rejuvenation.

These are powerful tools that not only improve your health and body, but will transform your daily outlook, your thoughts, and your relationships. But, like anything in life, consistency is the backbone for improvement. Tools are just tools until you show up.

Fortunately, from my experiences with strength training and fitness, I knew being part of a community helped make the process a lot more fun.

At Breakthrough Fitness, we've been able to create a winning combination of coaching, community and accountability. This combination is great for our clients in the gym, but what about the other 163+ hours of the week when our clients weren't with us?

That's where the articles in this book and hundreds of others come into play. They are my way of coaching from a distance, helping my clients and those that read them to stay the course and never stray too far from their fitness and health.

As you read these stories and lessons, you'll learn that "I walk with you". Each day, I have decisions to make and limiting beliefs to overcome. Alone, I struggle. Together, we rise up and live a healthy, robust life full of vitality.

Keep moving,

Coach Dom

ACCOMPLISHMENTS

t's really easy to get overwhelmed with fitness and living a healthier lifestyle. The amount of information and misinformation at your fingertips is endless. I'm sure you've read up on calorie burn, strength training and HIIT training. There's a good chance you read something about Keto and how carbs are the devil. You've been told you need more protein and that intermittent fasting could work along with everything else mysteriously popping up in your Facebook feed minutes after words leave your mouth.

Look, these things have merit, but none of them will keep you committed to your goals.

The driving force behind staying committed is the feeling of accomplishment. It's the most important aspect of fitness that no one ever mentions.

The daily victories of portion control, reducing alcohol, walking more often and doing a little strength training...

The accomplishment of turning off the alarm and putting workout clothes on. Now the big decision - do I get off the edge of this bed or listen to my voice listing the reasons I shouldn't?

The HUGE win at the edge of the bed reveals the path, which forks into many choices - private personal training facility, garage or home workout room, big box gym, running trail, yoga studio...

An hour later, you're alert and energized, ready to take on the day.

"Worked out" is now checked off the list!

This early victory leads to a healthy breakfast and positive vibes. You'll forget that the workout took place by noon, but the small, glorious victories that made it happen will have a powerful impact on your entire day.

Accomplishment is the most powerful weapon you have in your quest for a happier, healthier life.

Chapter One

THE 3 PRINCIPLES OF EXERCISE

L egendary football coach Vince Lombardi would begin every season with a speech to his team. He would say, "Men, this is football..." and then he would start breaking down the fundamentals of the sport.

Well folks, this is fitness and there are fundamental principles that we need to learn and follow.

The three principles (fundamental truths) are specificity, overload, and progression. It doesn't matter if you are strength training, running, or pole dancing. If you want to get results and continue to move forward, you need to stick to these principles.

Specificity

Simply put, you get what you train.

The exercise you choose should match what you are looking to accomplish. Let's say your biggest desire is to change the shape of your body. To do this, you'll need to change the way you eat and do physical activities that force the musculature of the entire body to work. Your body won't change with fresh air and good intentions. It needs a reason to change.

When most people think about changing the shape of their body, they think about losing weight. Now, losing weight can definitely be accomplished without exercise, but all you're really doing is making a smaller version of the same body.

The scale has changed and you may be smaller, but you can still have the same slumped shoulders, jiggly arms and squishy belly. Changing the actual shape of the body will require strength training and conditioning.

You'll have to lift weights. You can lift light weights and bodyweight for high repetitions (15+). You can lift moderate loads (weights) between 6-14 repetitions or you can lift heavier weights with low repetitions (3-5). Spending time in all three ranges is a smart choice.

You'll also need to move a lot (conditioning). You can walk, hike, ruck (walking or hiking with a weighted pack), swim, bike, row, run (preferably at different speeds and distances), do circuit training or play sports. The important thing is that you do something.

Overload

Pushing your body to do work it's not accustomed to doing. GET OUT OF YOUR COMFORT ZONE. I'll mention again that these principles apply to whatever you are doing. Coach Dan John said it best - intensity trumps volume.

Exercise needs to be intense. Let's continue to use weight loss (fat loss) as an example. Everyone gravitates towards running to lose fat. You run a mile and burn 100 calories in 15 minutes - just an example. You've gotten better at running that mile and now you are more efficient at using energy (calories). Don't get excited because efficiency means you are burning fewer calories to run that mile. You either have to go longer or faster to increase the intensity. Why would you want to run 20-30 minutes to burn the amount of calories it took in 15 minutes? How do you make it more intense? You go faster, run up a hill, or carry someone on your back.

You'll learn quickly though, that you can't always keep going further, faster or longer without diminishing returns.

Progression

Remember when fitness pole dancing was a thing? Let's say you got hooked on pole dancing and that's what you really enjoyed doing for fitness.

Do you remember how sore you were from swinging around the pole a few times? Your muscles never worked that way before. It felt great. You created a new stress, and the muscles responded. You even broke a nice sweat and burned a decent amount of calories. You're hooked!

As you continue to take classes, you get really good, but your body isn't responding as it once did. You need to step up your game and **progress** to more challenging moves. You begin climbing, flipping and spinning faster around the pole. Your friends chant, "go Jade, go, go, go Jade (your stage name of course) and you really turn up the intensity. The next day you are sore and really feel the extra work. That's because you stepped out of your comfort zone and created more stress that forced the body to adapt and eventually change. This is progression.

Those are the three principles of strength training and exercise. Make sure you are doing the appropriate stuff for your goal (specificity). Challenge yourself with the proper intensity (overload) and make sure to make steady progress.

Chapter Two

CONSISTENCY

I was getting a new client onboard yesterday and in our conversation she asked, "What do I need to do?"

I responded, "Well, you made the commitment to start, and that's a hard first step, so good job on that. Now it comes down to consistency, so what you need to do is just show up. Don't worry about what will take place in the gym, that's our responsibility. The only thing you need to focus on is showing up."

If you look at any area of your life that you consider successful, you'll see it's because you were consistent. Your actions were spot on sometimes and other times they weren't. You stuck your nose in there every day and got your fair share of bruises and you have the scars to prove it. You started from a position and worked your way up.

Body transformation, strength and life change aren't any different. It's a process that comes with victories and defeats.

One of the hardest things you'll have to do is manage compromises. Setting fitness and weight loss goals excludes options. This doesn't mean doing a lot of unsustainable things 100% of the time. All that will do is make you a grumpy pants. And no one enjoys being around a grumpy pants.

But you will need to reframe your perception of what's necessary and try to make things as simple as possible.

Exercising six days a week and never eating carbs is not sustainable for most of us. So, how can you reframe these goals?

- I will perform 1-2 strength workouts per week and 1-2 conditioning workouts (even if one or more of those workouts is at home, with the program prescribed by my coach).
- I will earn my carbs with exercise. (This means, eat a little more carbs in your meals following a workout, and a little less in all other meals during the day.)

For most people, following these two simple principles 80% of the time CONSISTENTLY will create a major transformation in 6-12 months.

My advice, if you choose to listen, is to pick a couple of things you can easily do EVERY WEEK and do those things EVERY WEEK. You may not reach your goals as fast as you like, but the possibility only remains if you never give up.

Chapter Three

WHAT IS SEMI-PRIVATE TRAINING

T he concept of personal training has changed a lot over the years. Between the years 1992-2009 I attended gyms. From 1992 to 1997 I attended Physiques Unlimited in Pompano Beach. Physiques was roughly a 3,000 square foot facility, filled with lots of stuff and mostly self-motivated people. The only personal trainer at this gym would move his clients from machine to machine, counting repetitions, giving a 'good job' occasionally. This was basically personal training in the mid-90's. It didn't seem like he did much, but the people he trained needed help. They needed an appointment and someone to dictate what they were going to do. They benefited from the movement and strength.

In 1999, I did my internship with a gentleman named Juan Carlos (JC) Santana in Boca Raton. JC was my first mentor, and he opened my eyes to a whole new style of training and coaching. He took training concepts that were being used in sports and rehabilitation and was one of the first few trainers who made 'functional training' mainstream.

During my internship, I helped JC train multiple clients at once. I remember throwing medicine balls with a client who had a brain injury and handicaps that made us think outside the box for his training. After throwing medicine balls with him, I would be coaching a 50-year-old client on deadlifts, always having my eye on a third client doing her training program. We were doing semi-private training, but we just called it training.

I also had the opportunity to be JC's assistant during functional training seminars for the National Strength and Conditioning Association, as well as visit a few collegiate strength and conditioning programs.

During the seminars, we coached dozens of aspiring fitness professionals in groups, teaching them functional training techniques using stability balls and other tools new to them.

In collegiate strength rooms, the team trained together.

When I finally decided to pursue personal training as a career in 2008, I had a vision of how I thought training should be done. My experiences shaped my vision.

- Training was always more fun and rewarding when I had a partner(s)
- The body is one piece.
- Free weights the majority of the time.
- The majority of training is completed while standing.

That year I met my next mentor, Alwyn Cosgrove, at a Perform Better conference.

Alywn and his wife Rachel have been running a successful facility in Santa Clarita, California. It was my exact vision - a personal training facility that provided clients with customized training programs, but coached them in a "semi-private" setting.

Fact - It's more fun to work out with other people. This can be a friend or a community of people looking to build strength and improve their fitness, just like you.

A semi-private training approach is much more cost-effective for the client, while still providing the individualized program and personal attention.

Here's how this might look in a 4-person session with clients at different stages of their fitness journey:

Client 1 is experienced with weightlifting and proficient with her movement, so she's following a program that includes barbell deadlifts and a high-intensity finisher.

Client 2 is similar to Client 1, but he has lower back issues. A trap bar deadlift is a safer option for him, and he'll finish his session with some mobility and flexibility work to support his lower back.

Clients 3 and 4 are a couple who just recently started training, so they'll be doing a circuit of bodyweight, resistance band and TRX exercises, with some core and corrective exercises to help build a strong foundation of quality movement.

All four people can enjoy training in the same environment, even though they are doing a program that is intelligently designed and appropriate for them.

Yes, personal training has changed... and I'd argue for the better.

Chapter Four

RANDOM THURSDAY NIGHT PIZZA

T here is at least one random night a week that I may not feel like cooking or the wife doesn't want what was planned. Since I'm the cook in the house, most of the burden for dinner falls on me. This is a good thing, because my wife's not a wonderful cook. In our house, when she cooks, we pray after we eat!

Let me paint a picture.....

It was a random Thursday. Before I left for work, I took chicken out of the freezer to thaw. Around 2pm I received the daily, "what are we doing for dinner" text from my wife. I replied, "I took chicken out." She replies with a screenshot of a Marco's Pizza advertisement and a big-eyed emoji.

Marco is a super nice guy. He always knows when to send us a postcard or drop us an email. He recently sent us this nice email.

Dear Dominic & Leslie,

We miss you! We haven't seen you for some time. We hope everything is okay. Dom, as you may know, the average American eats 23lbs of pizza each year. This means that a few of your neighbors are eating very little pizza and some are scarfing down more than 46lbs of pizza during a 365 day span. We are concerned that if you don't eat a pizza soon, you will not consume your 23lbs, falling below average. Dominic & Leslie, you know how much your old buddy Marco likes to hear from you, so if you call me today I'll give you a FREE 86 inch pizza when you purchase an 86 inch pizza. Please call today if you have the chance. I am really concerned.

Sincerely,

Marco

PS - Dial the 10 digits and the 2 liters are on us!

At this moment I had the power to say to my wife, "that's nice, but I already took out the chicken, so let's just eat that." Instead I replied, "I guess we can get pizza. Marco misses us."

Our decision snowballed.

My chicken dinner of roughly 400 calories was now well over 1,000 calories. No big deal, right? Until Friday comes along and our normal work/picking up children routine gets thrown for a loop. Next thing you know, we are sitting at Sonny's Real Pit BBQ for dinner! Chalk up another 1,000+ calorie meal, as well as throwing away chicken that went uncooked.

Who is going to say no?

Saying no would have eliminated one high calorie, fat bomb of a meal and kept money in our pocket. Instead,

I stuffed my face two nights in a row, feeling bloated and terrible.

Weight loss and weight management come down to choices. You can continue to hop from one fad diet to the next, losing and gaining the same pounds and then some.

Or you can take a reasonable, sustainable approach by reducing or eliminating random Thursday night pizza, Wednesday night White Claws or cutting out snacks during your Bridgerton binge.

It's your choice.

Chapter Five

DEFINE FIT

R eal success isn't just reaching your goal, but also sustaining it. For this to happen, we need a plan and a little legwork. After that, it comes down to TAKING ACTION!

I think your fitness and health plan starts with your definition of 'fit'.

Think about your "why". Maybe it's keeping up with your kids or being healthy and active when you are a grandparent. Your "why" could be to maintain energy levels, immune health and strength into your 70s and 80s.

You need to dig really deep to find a purpose for living a healthy, active life.

Define "Fit"

- What is considered "Fit" by me might differ completely for you.
- Don't fall into a trap that you need to train or look a certain way.
- This is all about you, nobody else.
- Fitness is just one part of your life.

- Your definition will change over the course of your life.

Here is my definition of fit:

My Why's....

- Be a role model to my children, so they can learn that eating well and exercise is part of a vibrant life.
- I want to possess the ability to apply strength, run quickly and be agile enough to handle myself in an unexpected situation.
- Live a robust, high-quality life until I die.

Now that I have purpose, I can devise a plan

- Challenge myself with purposeful strength and hypertrophy training 3-4x per week. This type of training provides the biggest return on my investment of time.
- Incorporate activities and workouts that focus on athleticism, conditioning and muscular endurance.
- Spend most of my time standing and moving, not sitting. I'm currently looking into a stand-up desk for when I'm working on the computer.
- Keeping my weight around 180ish and body fat below 15%. These numbers help me create boundaries, which will require me to have a weekly meal plan, drink less alcohol, reduce processed foods, increase vegetables and be more mindful of my choices.
- Be pain-free - Listen to my body and don't force workouts and make time each day to work on keeping the joints and muscles loose.
- Spend more time outdoors doing leisure activities.

- Demonstrate discipline, so I have the freedom to enjoy the foods and drinks that I want when I want.

Now it's your turn. A clear definition will help you create a plan. Don't make it too rigid. A good plan is flexible. Get started, don't stop and adjust the plan as needed.

Chapter Six

4 REASONS WHY YOU MAY NOT BE LOSING WEIGHT

L et's get straight to the point. Losing weight requires a calorie deficit. Calories In vs. Calories Out (CICO) matters.

Creating a deficit consistently until the weight is off isn't easy. It will take a lot of preparation and work, but you can do it.

Here are 4 things you need to have an honest assessment about because they may hinder your progress.

1. Weekend overeating

Calories still matter on the weekend. I know many people have a "cheat meal/day". This can work on a fat loss plan, but you still have to understand how it affects your weekly caloric budget.

Food labels and restaurant menus aren't totally accurate when it comes to nutritional facts. They aren't even legally bound to provide accuracy. Dinner out on Friday and takeout lunch on Saturday can easily add hundreds if not thousands of additional calories.

Try using a food tracking app on your phone for a couple of weeks. This experience can provide you with valuable data on where your additional calories may come from.

2. Untracked alcohol

I had a couple of drinks... did you have two? Or did you have 5?

If you are a drinker, you know how easily a glass of wine can become a bottle. Your 100 calorie White Claws add up quickly.

Also, we can easily lose sight of portion control and snacking when the buzz kicks in.

It's not just the calories. The effects of alcohol on hormones and metabolism can work against your fat loss efforts.

3. Underestimating food intake/calories

As I mentioned above, food labels and menus can be inaccurate.

We also forget about the pat of butter on our toast or how we eye-balled the tablespoon of oil the recipe called for.

How much cheese is the actual "sprinkle" on your salad or eggs?

And let's not forget about that big ole scoop of peanut butter or heavy pour of coffee creamer.

There is research that shows people actually underestimate their caloric intake by 50%!

Dressings, sauces and fat from oils and butter are very, very sneaky.

4. Overestimated activity

I love to eat, just like most of my clients. BUT, as the saying goes... YOU WILL NOT OUT-TRAIN A POOR DIET.

Exercise for many people isn't about the feeling of accomplishment and happy endorphins. It's about calories burned. You rely on your watch or some other technology that tells you how you've burned an insane amount of calories per day. Those monitors and devices have been shown to overestimate calories burned by 30-90%!

So, as an example, your device is saying 1,000 calories, but that could be 700 or less.

If you are serious about fat loss, the best thing is to track and weigh everything you eat for the next two weeks. This will be an eye-opening experience and will change the way you eat.

Also weigh yourself every day at the same time, under the same conditions. Keep track of your average weekly weight and your average weekly calorie intake. You'll get a good idea of what's really going on by doing this.

This isn't something you have to do forever, but it's a great way to create awareness. For losing fat and keeping it off, mindfulness and awareness of what, how, where and with whom we eat are foundational elements that must be in place.

Don't look at this list and get overwhelmed because all four hit a nerve. Choose one and work on it. One change can go a very long way.

Chapter Seven

MOMENTUM

One of the oldest sports cliches has to do with which team has the "momentum."

And it's funny, the team that's winning always seems to have the momentum, if you ask the "analysts." And the team that's losing doesn't have any at all.

The reality is that both teams have momentum.

The winning team is moving forward positively.

The losing team is simply going the wrong way at the moment.

But, momentum can change quickly in sports....

And in fitness and health.

Momentum comes from action and, unfortunately, inaction. So if you're in a groove with consistent workouts, getting plenty of sleep and prepping your healthy meals, you've got momentum.

And if you picked up the habit of drinking nightly or snacking, you too have momentum.

Momentum can be a double-edged sword because it will keep going as long as the actions that cause it to continue to happen.

In football, if things are not going the right way, you make adjustments. Maybe it's a different play or a new defensive formation that will get executed better.

Next thing you know, momentum has changed.

Just remember that regardless of which way the momentum is going for you at the moment, you have the ability to either keep it going or change it.

The choice is yours.

Chapter Eight

LASTING CHANGE

Yesterday (Tuesday), I started the day off with a nice breakfast of eggs, sliced avocado, and fruit before heading to Breakthrough Fitness. After five steady hours of training clients, I was starving. I grabbed my bag, my container of chicken tortilla soup, and was getting in my car to head home for lunch.

As I started the car, I looked over at my chicken tortilla soup with disgust. "I've been eating you since Sunday dinner. I'm done with your ass". Unhealthy Dom has gained control of my thoughts, while Healthy Dom pleaded from the backseat to "just eat the soup".

We went back and forth considering nuggets and Polynesian sauce from Chick-fil-a, fried chicken from Popeyes, a burrito from Moe's or a burger from Burger Fi. All sounded far more delicious than three-day-old chicken tortilla soup.

A decision had to be made. Turn right out of Breakthrough Fitness and Unhealthy Dom wins. Turn left, get home and Healthy Dom has a chance. At that very moment, I remembered the sliced ham and cheese that Ben loved last week, but wants nothing to do with this week. Five-year-old's...

Still hangry, I warmed up my soup and made a hot ham and cheese on rye bread, which sparked interest from my son. Unhealthy Dom finally stopped bitching and began enjoying the soup and sandwich. He even gave half to Ben.

My decision was a victory. My half sandwich and soup were roughly 500 calories, with about 15 grams of protein. Yes, I also had bread and dairy, which some people would have you believe are handcrafted in hell by the devil himself. Forgive me, lord for I have sinned.

What I didn't have was a 1,000 plus calorie lunch loaded with fat that would have left me feeling bloated and lethargic.

How many times a week are you faced with a decision like this?

One reasonable decision each week could save you 26,000 calories a year.

What if you went one night without the 150 calories from the wine or small treat?

There's another 7,800.

We build lasting change on good decisions made daily.

Chapter Nine

4 REASONS TO HIRE A PERSONAL TRAINER

Dedicating time to strength training and fitness can be difficult, especially if it's never been part of your life. Maybe the idea of hiring a personal trainer has crossed your mind.

Here are four situations that may warrant an expert with knowledge on program design, exercise selection, and nutritional foundations.

1. If You're New To Strength Training Or Working Out In General

When you're at the beginning stages of fitness, you have a lot of questions and things to learn.

How often should I go... how long should I be spending at the gym... what should I do first... should I be eating carbs or not... should I be using the machines or free weights...

For a beginner, this can be a challenge. And one thing I've learned from coaching hundreds of clients is that most people don't want to think.

The additional stress of trying to figure out fitness on your own, when you already have plenty of life stress, doesn't work. Hiring a trainer (if they're good) will divorce you from the responsibility of training. You just need to show up.

A good coach is going to build a program based on your abilities and goals. If they do their job well, you'll properly progress through exercises, learning by doing. A coach accelerates the learning curve, helps you avoid common mistakes, and is always teaching.

2. You're Bored

Coach Dom's golden rules to exercise:

- Do something.
- Do something you like.

If you don't enjoy jogging, don't jog because you'll eventually quit.

Hiring a trainer can prevent boredom by keeping your workouts challenging by changing up your routine. My coaching philosophy is "same, but different." It's my job to make the basics fun and fresh, so you continue to do them. This variety can help you break through plateaus, but most importantly, it keeps you coming back again and again.

You won't get strong, lean, fit, and happy without coming back again and again and again....

3. You've Stopped Seeing Results

Results and improvements keep us driven. When you've been exercising for quite some time, improvements don't come as they once did. The majority of the time, you don't need to ditch your program. A good coach can evaluate your workout routine and make subtle changes that will get you over the hump. A short-term investment with a coach can help you tighten up form and intensity during your sessions, which will pay big dividends.

4. You Need Support & Accountability

Fitness is a process. Becoming stronger, leaner, and happier requires time and effort. That effort has to be hard enough to elicit change. They'll be days you conspire with the universe, trying to find something, anything that would be a better option than your workout. The snooze button will have its victories.

We all need support and accountability to grow and improve. Enter a professional coach.

A coach brings a lot to the table -knowledge, attitude, energy, passion, personality... and these qualities are powerful tools that will help provide you the support you need.

You know what else is powerful?

An appointment.

Having to be somewhere at a particular place and time with a professional who's passionate about helping you is extremely powerful. An appointment, an excellent coach that you like and a training environment you feel comfortable in, is a winning combination.

You are also making a financial commitment when hiring a professional. You'll get a glorious return on your investment if you show up and trust your coach.

If you've been on the fence about hiring a trainer, then these four reasons can push you in the right direction.

A coach is a person in your corner, not an expensive piece of equipment in the corner.

A coach is someone who believes in you. That belief comes in handy, especially when you may not yet believe in yourself. A coach can provide valuable feedback and help you see things from a new perspective.

If you're a beginner or you just want to tackle a new challenge, then your first item of business should be to hire a professional trainer to make sure you're on the right path.

Chapter Ten

THE GOLDEN RULES

There are two golden rules of exercise. They are:

#1 - Do something you enjoy.

#2 - Do something else.

Let's look at all the movement you do in a week and divide it up into buckets.

Strength training bucket

- Structured workouts lifting weights to build, tone and change the shape of your body.

Interval training/circuit training bucket

- A combination of high, moderate and low-intensity periods of exercise. Could be a specific type of exercise like running or a combination of bodyweight exercises, light weights, calisthenics and cardio - bike, row, run, etc.
- Group training classes, boot camps.
- Emphasis is on muscular endurance and conditioning.

Mobility and flow bucket

- Yoga, Pilates, barre, stretch routines.

- Emphasis on stability, flexibility, isometric and bodyweight strength (relative strength)

Steady-state cardio bucket

- Jogging, biking, speed walking...
- Heart rate stays elevated for the duration of the workout.
- Duration determines intensity.

Physical recreation

- Walking, playing sports, bowling league, martial arts, pickle ball.

Daily movement

- At work
- At home before leaving for work and when you get back home.
- Chores, etc.

Now tell me, what bucket is overflowing?

Which ones have a little movement in them?

Which ones are completely empty?

Most people who dedicate time to fitness usually gravitate towards a specific style of training. Runners run and do nothing else. People lift weights for strength and body composition, but never stretch or condition the heart and lungs.

I'm a genuine believer that movement is the engine that drives vitality, so I think it's great that you have a full bucket.

But, the repetition of only one kind of movement may lead to aches, pains and injuries.

The best thing we can do for quality of life is to take a little out of our full bucket and do something else.

Runners would benefit by adding to their strength bucket. The mobility and flow bucket compliments strength training and Interval training rather nicely.

If all your buckets are currently empty, start increasing daily movement and physical recreation. I would also consider hiring a fitness coach and learn how to properly strength train.

If all you do is one thing, then I recommend giving up a day of that (you won't make or find more time) and do something else. Your mind and body will love you for it.

Chapter Eleven

BACK ON TRACK

There's one phrase I've heard more often than almost anything else I can think of when speaking with people about their fitness plan.

"I need to get back on track."

What does this mean?

Our track is our track, and we're always on it. The habits and action steps we follow daily determine whether we're moving forward on that track, standing still, or going backwards.

How do you ensure that you're always moving forward?

You start by ditching the "all or nothing" mindset.

If you hit a rough period with your schedule, whether that's work, school, kids or all of the above, there's a temptation to give up or "pause" your fitness program. This belief comes from the "all or nothing" mindset.

How can you break this pattern?

Stop trying to be perfect.

Stop believing that if you don't have time for a gym workout and healthy meals that support your weight loss or body composition goals, it's a lost day.

It's not.

There is always ONE thing you can do (or not do) that will move you closer to your goals.

Control what you can control. No time to get to the gym? Get some movement in at home and hit your water intake goal for the day (which takes no extra time, by the way).

You could also ask for help. Having a coach or even just a workout buddy can go a long way toward helping you stay accountable. They can also help you not get discouraged when things don't go as planned. And things will definitely not always go as planned.

Remember, there is no such thing as being "on track" or "off track." We're ALWAYS on track. It is just a question of whether we are moving and in what direction.

Chapter Twelve

BLOWN TIRE SYNDROME

A nother work week is in the books and you've stuck to your nutrition and exercise plan all week. You ate breakfast every day, packed a healthy lunch and snacks, and made it to the gym four times. You even scheduled a Saturday bike ride with some friends. You're feeling good about the week, so you join a few coworkers for happy hour. You know it's going to be okay because you're "just going to have one".

The first drink hits your lips, and the unwinding begins. Jokes are being told and good times are being had. Someone orders a couple of appetizers, because they're ravenously hungry. They didn't plan like you, so they haven't eaten since breakfast. You're not really hungry, but the one Moscow Mule has already become two. The alcohol has increased your appetite, so you decide to grab a chip and start to dip. Damn, the chip broke as you were trying to scoop that hunk of artichoke. It's rude to leave half a chip in the bowl, so without thinking, you scoop again. This time you were so successful, you kept going as if you were on a roll at the craps table. Oh snap, you got some on your knuckle. You've officially blown a tire and veered off your nutrition plan.

What the hell? Who ordered these shots? There goes your testosterone production along with tire number two.

You somehow managed to get out with two tires intact. Now you're starving and you begin to search for cheap, convenient prey. Your choices are bountiful as their bright signs light up the night's sky, beckoning you with the scents of greasy flesh and salty goodness. It calls to you, 'your precious' and your willpower crumbles like crispy bacon. Mmmmmm, bacon!

You pull into your driveway on your unicycle: tread worn thin, air slowly seeping out of the last tire. You get a call from a friend who is having a barbecue tomorrow. Pop! Tire four bursts. You text your friends, canceling your bike ride, waving goodbye to all the hard work you put in during the week. Pass the Sangria and let's get this fiesta started! Vamanos!

We all blow tires. Stopping and fixing the tire will determine how successful you are at fat loss and weight management.

Chapter Thirteen

BE THE BOSS

O n the weekends, it's rare that I don't have music playing. Growing up, my parents exposed me to all genres of music and I'll do the same with my kids. Right now they're getting a healthy dose of rock, pop and r&b from all decades. Someday, when I'm not concerned with exposing them to explicit lyrics, they'll get the full arsenal of 90s Gansta Rap and Hip Hop from the 2000s.

In the meantime, it's family friendly like the Michael Jackson Essentials playlist on Apple Music. We jammed to hit after hit - Billy Jean, Beat it, PYT, The Way You Make Me Feel...

And then Man in the Mirror came on and made me think about today's email.

YOU are the BOSS of your life. The CEO.

Let that sink in.

By my own unscientific estimate, about 99% of the problems we have in our life come from one person. The one we see in the mirror each day.

YOU are the CEO of your life in every area. For better or worse, you are the technician, the manager, the accountant, the VP, the CFO, and ultimately, the CEO of everything.

YOU are the CEO of your eating. You and you alone are responsible for the things you eat and put into your body (and your children).

YOU are the CEO of your fitness. You and you alone decide to work out or not, to skip the training session or attend it. You decide to give today's 100% or go through the motions.

YOU are the CEO of your attitude. You and you alone decide to wake up in a good mood each day (or not). You decide to take things in stride (or get sidetracked by them). You decide to see the glass as half-full or half-empty.

YOU are the CEO of every situation, problem, and event you encounter in this life. You can't control what happens to you, but you are 100% in control of your thoughts about those situations and how you react to them.

YOU are the boss. You are in complete control of your life. And thus, you are 100% responsible for the outcomes you've received until this point.

Are you happy with them? Great, keep doing you!

If you're not, it's time to take ownership and start working on happiness.

Now is a perfect time to start.

Chapter Fourteen

THE BEST AND WORST FAT LOSS PROGRAM

Everyone wants immediate results, and they wanted them yesterday. That's why I came up with the following program. I was inspired while driving home and saw a sign posted outside our local sod farm - Sod Stacker Wanted.

My first thought was, "This is it! My big program that will put me in the upper echelon of trainers." You know, people like Jillian Michaels and Suzanne Somers. My second thought was, "If I were trying to lose fat fast, sod stacking would be the way to go." My third thought was, "Our members would all be in amazing shape if I could get them to do my Sod Stacker Insanity Program."

The program would be:

- Wake up, eat protein and vegetables.
- Stack sod outside for four hours.
- Take a thirty-minute break to eat more protein, berries and nuts.
- Stack sod for four more hours.
- Go home and eat protein and vegetables.Shower.
- Sleep.

Do this same routine for the next 5 days. Then take the weekend off.

Pros vs. cons of the Sod Stacker Insanity Program

Pros

- Sod stacking doesn't require any equipment. If you don't have access to sod, you can use bricks, sandbags or whatever materials you have that can be stacked.
- Sod stacking requires musculature of the entire body, making it a fantastic "big bang for your buck" movement for fat loss.
- Sod stacking can be learned quickly. Simply bend down, grab a few pieces of sod and stack it.

Cons

- Sod Stacker Insanity requires eight hours of commitment a day, five days a week.
- Sod stacking isn't much fun.

Time commitment and enjoyment of the process are two critical factors that need to be determined prior to beginning a training program. Sod Stacking, along with many activities, can lead to fat loss, but at what cost?

This would be the small print at the bottom of the infomercial for Sod Stacker Insanity - *some symptoms of The Sod Stacker Insanity and The Sod Stacker Insanity x infinity can be, but are not limited to: Anger, grumpiness, skin cancer, boredom, missing your children grow up, divorce.....*

If you aren't enjoying the process, the program is not sustainable. If a program requires an eight-hour commitment and you only have three to four, then it's not sensible.

Doing something repetitively leads to change. Your ultimate rewards (losing fat, building strength, dropping inches) will come from when you do something repetitively with the proper intensity for as often as you can commit to doing it. Whatever you decide to do, make sure it's sensible and sustainable.

Chapter Fifteen

BREAKING BAD

It's easy to convince ourselves that massive success requires massive action. The reality is that improving by 1% may not be noticeable, but it can be far more meaningful, especially in the long run.

Success is the product of daily habits, not once in-a-lifetime transformations.

So, it doesn't really matter where you are at right now with your health and fitness. What matters is whether your habits are putting you on the right path towards your goals.

Focus on your current trajectory rather than your current results.

Imagine you have an ice cube sitting at the table in front of you. The room is a cold, 25 degrees. Ever so slowly, the room begins to heat up.

26 degrees.

27 degrees.

28 degrees.

Nothing has changed.

29 degrees.

30 degrees

31 degrees

Still, nothing has happened.

Then, 32 degrees. The ice begins to melt.

A one degree shift, seemingly no different from the temperature increases before it, has unlocked an enormous change.

During any quest, there is often a "Valley of Disappointment." We expect to see results fast. We want the scale to go down immediately because we made some changes to our nutrition and added in a little movement. It's easy to get frustrated and feel you aren't making progress when you see little change over the first few days, weeks, and even months.

Once this kind of thinking takes over, it's easy to let good habits fall by the wayside.

This is when good habits have to persist.

Your work was not wasted; it's just being stored.

Like the ice cube, change is taking place.

Keep striving for 1% better and your breakthrough moment will happen.

Chapter Sixteen

SIMPLE TIPS FOR HEALTHY EATING ON A BUDGET

A ll too often I hear people say eating healthy is expensive.

I disagree. Yes, if you are buying grass-fed beef, fresh wild-caught fish and organic chicken, your grocery bill will definitely be higher.

However, eating right and including healthy foods doesn't have to break the bank.

If you follow these tips, you'll eat healthy and make it fit into your weekly grocery budget.

1. Plan Your Meals

- Meal planning will do wonders for your diet and your wallet.
- When you meal plan, you shop with a list. You need to get what's on the list and get out. Snaking up and down the aisles will surely lead to temptation and impulse purchases.
- Be sure to take an inventory of what you already have. It's easy to buy duplicate items that you already have on hand. This could drive up your grocery bill.

2. Buy in bulk, take advantage of sales

- You can buy a $2.39 box of rice pilaf that feeds your family one dinner, or you can buy a 16oz bag of brown rice for $1.15 that will provide you 4 full cups of uncooked rice... that's a lot of rice!

And you can try this easy rice pilaf recipe!

https://www.spendwithpennies.com/easy-rice-pilaf/

- Meats - buy whole chickens and cut them up yourself. You can also buy skin-on/bone-in chicken. You have to do the prep work, but it saves money. Chicken thighs are less expensive than breasts and can be trimmed of additional fat.
- Take advantage when chicken and pork are BOGO.
- Beans, rice, potatoes, and eggs are inexpensive.
- I love Costco! I can get a 12-pack of canned organic black beans for less than $.70 cents a can. I can also get things like frozen, vacuum sealed, wild-caught fish and $5 rotisserie chickens.

3. Avoid Takeout

We had Bolay for dinner the other night. The meal was healthy, but we spent close to $40 on this one meal (me, wife, kids - 8- and 5-year-old).

If we get takeout once a week, that's $160 easy for the month. How many fruits and veggies can you buy for $160?

Eating more meals at home is a wise choice for your pocketbook and your waistline.

4. Save Leftovers For Lunch

If you want to save on both time and money, cooking extra is the right move.

By making larger meals, you can save the extra for lunch the next day or you can freeze and save it for later.

Using leftovers is great for your health and your budget.

5. Don't Shop Hungry

How many times have you done your grocery shopping while hungry? I did it this past weekend and ended up with a block of cheese and a box of crackers that weren't on the list. The ice cream was on the list in my eight-year-old daughter's handwriting, but that's another story.

Shopping while hungry will make you stray from your list, therefore adding items that may not be healthy, and that may be more expensive. This could tank your budget fast. Always make sure you're shopping on a full stomach to prevent impulse buys, so you can focus on keeping your health and weight loss on track.

Follow these tips and eat healthy while staying within your budget.

Chapter Seventeen

THE FOUNDATIONAL THREE

Olivia (my 8-year-old) has started gymnastics. She likes it, pays attention and wants to learn - three things necessary for getting better at anything in life.

Want to improve your marriage?

- You need to like the person you are married to.
- Pay attention to them.
- Learn how to communicate better.

Want to improve your fitness and health?

- Pick something you enjoy.
- Pay attention to what you put in your mouth.
- Learn how to strengthen and condition your body properly.

Now back to the story...

Olivia is learning the basic tumbling moves - forward roll, back bend, cartwheel, bridge. These are called the fundamentals and until they're mastered, you can't really do much else in gymnastics.

Learning how to squat, properly, bend (hinge) properly and create full body tension (maybe the most important) are fundamentals of strength training.

What is full body tension? Put a heavy item in your left hand and stand upright. Pay attention to how the body tightens up to resist the object from pulling you to the left. Feel how taunt the muscles get on your right side. That's tension.

I just described what we call a suitcase carry. Essentially, it's a walking side plank. Tension helps us learn that the body is one piece. The more you deliberately train tension, the more you'll pay attention to it when it's needed in real life... You'll automatically brace and tighten when picking up and moving bags of mulch all day. A strong torso (pillar) that has been programmed to engage and stabilize will allow you to play chicken in the pool with your kids without throwing your back out.. That same pillar of strength will help you be the grandparent that can handle three days of non-stop movement and fun when you visit the grandkids. You didn't expect a relaxing vacation, did you?

Homework...

Every day do some variation of a plank and/or carry. Remember, push-ups are a moving plank, which makes them a pleasant choice. Don't just go through the motions. Focus and feel where the tension needs to be. You'll learn a lot about your body.

I wouldn't hold a plank any longer than two minutes, but I would find ways to make the plank more challenging. You make carries more challenging by increasing the load.

Chapter Eighteen

WORKPLACE DILEMMA

L unch should just be a meal in the middle of the day that provides us nourishment and keeps us energized for the rest of the day. Depending on your work environment, lunch can often be a metabolism smoldering, blood-sugar spiking, nap time at your desk taking, artery clogging, muffin top materializing, pants unbuttoning, chicken-parm-you-taste-so-good, poor decision.

Workplace war zone

The workplace is like a war zone when you are trying to eat well and live healthy. You walk in the front door and wonder if Big Sal is going to keep his consecutive streak of showing up with donuts going. Yep, he did! Then there are the candy bowls that are like IEDs (improvised explosive devices) for your diet. Oh, what's that? It's someone's birthday again. Woopty-doo! Let's celebrate another grown ass man's 46th birthday with sweets. I haven't even got to the worst culprit of all - lunch!

The Drawer of menus

The drawer has all the usual suspects: Italian, Chinese, subs, burritos, barbecue and various restaurants. Every day, the drawer gets opened and someone places the call for pickup or delivery. The only person safe is the one who, from day one, has brought their own lunch. The person who has it the toughest is the one trying to make a change. When you try to break out of the lunch group, you'll get ridiculed, teased, and made to feel like an outsider. It's the crabs in a bucket syndrome.

Crabs in a Bucket Syndrome - When a bunch of crabs are placed in a bucket, none of them will get out. As one crab tries to climb out of the bucket, another crab will reach up and pull them back down.

How to succeed at eating healthy at work when no one else cares

Step 1 - Realize that nobody cares

Your health and fitness are your own personal responsibility. Your co-workers (who do not care about making a change) will hate the fact that you are trying. They will be even more angry because of your success. Don't take it personal. It has nothing to do with you and everything to do with them.

Step 2 - Partner up with the coworker who has already been making the choices you want to make

You need an ally because success is a team sport. More importantly, this person can be a mentor or someone to lean on for advice and accountability. This person may not exist in your workplace. I'm sure someone else wants to make the same changes. They're just too nervous to start. Find that person and form a team.

Step 3- Bring your own lunch

Leftovers of last night's dinner work well. A salad with protein is great too. If you have an office with a good break room, maybe a smoothie. Lunch shouldn't be a tremendous ordeal.

Step 4 - Stand up for yourself

Make it clear to your co-workers what you are doing. Most will respect your decisions if you put it out there. Your actions will dictate what happens next. If your actions do the talking, I bet you'll end up with a few people interested in what you are doing. Success often leads to a leadership position. Be ready for it and embrace it.

Step 5 - Get out of the building

I don't know how long you get for lunch, but if you get an hour, eat your food and then go for a walk. I know you have deadlines and work to do, but it isn't going anywhere. That thirty-minute walk will be the best part of your workday. You'll burn some calories, loosen up the joints and relax the mind, which will lead to better productivity.

The workplace dilemma can be a genuine struggle. I've had members drop substantial weight and improve their health and fitness by tackling this one challenge. It won't be easy, but if you truly have a desire to change, you'll do it.

Chapter Nineteen

THE SCALE, FRIEND OR FOE

S cale - a device used to measure mass.

The bathroom scale - a device designed to mentally torture humans every morning by getting them to stand on it and then showing them a number.

Of all the good indicators of health and fitness, we choose a number on a device that only measures total mass.

It doesn't measure how much of that mass is muscle, bone and organs vs. how much is fat (unless it's a real fancy scale).

It doesn't tell you about your resting heart rate or blood pressure. It knows nothing about stress or hydration levels or how well you slept last night.

It doesn't tell you your cholesterol, much less how much of your cholesterol is HDL (good) vs. LDL (bad).

The scale is probably the single least informative indicator of your current state of your health and fitness, yet every morning you'll shuffle to the bathroom and get on that device buck naked because every ounce matters.

If this one-dimensional snapshot every morning determines whether you're succeeding or failing at living a healthy, active life, then the scale is a FOE.

The scale is your FRIEND if it's part of a multi-dimensional snapshot consisting of how well your clothes fit, waist and hip measurements, photos, mood, energy levels, sleep quality and, most importantly, overall happiness.

Personally, I like the scale to be more of an acquaintance than a close friend. Someone that you are cool with, but only see at your friends' kids' birthday parties a few times a year.

Chapter Twenty

THE DIFFERENCE MAKER

It was probably ten years ago that I attended a strength and conditioning clinic at the University of Florida. Mick Marotti, then head football strength coach, was describing the culture of the weight room and how there is **no substitute for effort**. This is a guy who has been in the business of getting athletes stronger and faster for 28 years. The exercise programs are only as good as the effort being put forth.

I can give two people with identical fitness levels the same program and the one who gives more effort will get better results. Muhammad Ali hated training, but he loved being a champion. The only way he was going to be champion was by giving maximum effort in his training.

Effort is not a talent, it's a mindset

I heard it put this way by Jim Wendler, a world-class power lifter and strength coach. A good coach can get more out of you. Training with others can push you to work harder.

A positive training environment is a must and will encourage effort, but it all starts with you.

Eating well is not a talent, it's a mindset.

Hands down, the hardest part for most of us is changing our eating habits. The person who gives more effort eats better. It has nothing to do with willpower or discipline.

When I was in college, I knew how to cook eggs, boil rice, brown meat, make tuna salad and cook chicken on my George Foreman grill. I would also make a batch of Silly Chili that took me 15 minutes to make. It comprised browning ground beef, draining beef, opening a can of kidney beans, dumping beans into beef and sprinkling chili powder, salt and pepper. Very gourmet. I created my mindset from my goal of wanting to pack on muscle. To do that, I needed to eat an abundance of food. It didn't require me to be a chef, but it required effort.

Nowadays, life is busy, and I have mouths to feed. More effort is required for eating healthy the majority of the time. Now I have to look at my calendar, my wife's schedule, the kids' activities and so forth. When effort meets the calendar, we eat well. When we slack on effort (which we do) we don't eat as well.

What if you gave 1% more effort towards one or a few of these things: meal planning, preparation, keeping trigger foods out of the house, cooking, eating slowly, not being excessive when you eat snacks or drink alcohol, eating one additional serving of vegetables, stop eating when you are 80% full...

What if you gave 1% more effort during your workouts, mobility, stretching and low-intensity movement like walking...

What if you gave 1% more effort towards doing things that make you happy?

Chapter Twenty-one

LOOSE HABITS, TIGHT PANTS

I recently spent ten days in the Florida Keys. That's 10 days of loose nutrition habits.

We pulled back into town on Sunday afternoon.

Being gone so long, we had a bunch of things to do, so the easiest solution for dinner was takeout.

But takeout would have continued the madness of high calorie meals that affect my mood and energy. I wanted to start the week feeling good. That Sunday night dinner was an important meal. It needed to consist of foods that leave me feeling good.

Food that makes me feel good

I like my nutrition to revolve around these foods each week:

- Broccoli
- Green beans
- Mushrooms
- Onions
- Rice
- Avocado
- Eggs

- Fruit - the type of fruit varies, but right now it's berries, banana, apples and watermelon.
- Meat - chicken, pork, fish, beef.
- Beans

These items create the foundation for my weekly meals.

- None of these foods leave me feeling bloated and uncomfortable.
- It's hard for me to overeat these foods (even if I do, I don't feel bad).
- I feel mentally sharp and energized from these foods.

From here, I come up with a meal plan. That might be eggs with a piece of rye toast or chicken with mushrooms, onions and rice (my dinner on Sunday night). There are plenty of other foods in my diet, but I never have a bad week of nutrition when I start with my Big Ten.

When my meals are built around these foods, I don't need to worry about calories. I simply focus on two things:

- Eating slowly and mindfully
- Portions

Give this approach to nutrition a try. Create a list of 10 whole foods (minimally processed) that you enjoy and leave you feeling good.

Chapter Twenty-two

THE FOUNTAIN OF YOUTH – STRENGTH TRAINING

- Be aware of your oils and butter when cooking.
- Focus on portion sizes and eating at a slow pace.
- Pay attention to what you are eating when you aren't sitting down for a meal (snacks, random things).
- Ask yourself, how can I make this meal better?

S trength training is quality of life insurance.

Every aspect of fitness improves with strength. Mobility and joint health improves when you perform the basic fundamental movements you were born to do - squat, bend, push, pull and carry things. Your balance and ability to stabilize and resist injury gets better with strength. Your ability to stand upright with good posture and handle your daily activities improves with strength.

"Coach, isn't weightlifting dangerous? I don't want to get injured."

Being weak is dangerous and the culprit for most injuries. Lifting weights with proper form and the appropriate intensity for your abilities is very safe.

"But coach, I don't want to get bulky."

The easiest way to a bulky physique is the combination of a sedentary lifestyle, poor sleep, high stress and the consumption of too much energy (calories).

If you DO NOT want to build big, thick muscles, you won't. Big, thick muscles require lots of intense training, large quantities of food and a burning desire to do so.

"I just want to lose weight, so why do I need strength training?"

Lean mass (muscle) and activity play a huge role in how our body digests, absorbs and utilizes nutrients. Simply put, muscle and movement are necessary for losing fat, but more importantly, keeping it off for good. Also, strength is one of the most important indicators of health and longevity as we age. This makes resistance training a very important part of your fitness portfolio.

Strength training is the Fountain of Youth. The magic elixir that flows from the fountain is invigorating. You can build a robust body by visiting the fountain a few times a week. A little goes a long way.

Strength training is an investment that pays extraordinary dividends. It's never too late to invest in yourself. Commit a few hours a week, hire a coach, and enjoy the vitality and vigor that comes from your dedication.

Chapter Twenty-three

WHAT IS CIRCUIT TRAINING?

W hat is circuit training?

I define circuit training as interval strength training. I also like the term "cardio-strength training", which I first heard from Coach Robert Dos Remedios. A circuit is a sequence of exercises where the client moves from exercise to exercise in a predetermined sequence. At each exercise station, the client will do a certain amount of repetitions or do the exercise for a specific amount of time before moving to the next station. Between stations, there can be rest periods or it can be a continuous circuit.

Why circuit training?

- Very effective at raising work capacity (conditioning).
- Great for changing body composition.
- Can be tailored to target specific areas of the body.
- Team or group training can be performed safely with a large number of participants.
- Can be designed to address all aspects of fitness-strength, balance, agility, endurance... It is a very versatile training method.

- A circuit can have built in regressions or progressions for each exercise, allowing all levels of fitness to work together.
- Great for people with minimal time to train. You can get a lot of work done in a short time.
- Can be done with no equipment or all the training tools you have at your disposal - dumbbells, bands, balls, barbells...

Circuit training do's and don'ts

- The exercises must be strenuous. The work can't be too easy. Now don't read this, as you need to be crushed by the training session. What I'm saying is you should feel like you worked your body hard.
- I prefer keeping the exercises simple. When you get fatigued, your form will break down, which may lead to injury.
- Understand the flow of the circuit. You need to know what you want out of the circuit when you design it.

Criteria for circuits

Time

- Doing each exercise for a prescribed amount of time.

Repetitions

- You can do a repetition-based circuit where you do each exercise for a specific amount of t

Rest

- Rest between each exercise in a circuit.

- Rest between rounds of a circuit - A round is a completion of all exercises in a circuit.

Here is a four exercise circuit as an example:

Each exercise gets performed for 30 seconds, followed by a 15 second rest. After you complete all four exercises, take a 60 second rest. Repeat circuit.

Push-ups x 30 seconds

Rest 15 seconds

Sit-ups x 30 seconds

Rest 15 seconds

Squats x 30 seconds

Rest 15 seconds

Mountain climbers x 30 seconds

Rest 60 seconds

Circuit training for the win!

For overall fitness, circuit training is a fun, challenging way to train. Bodyweight or any implement you desire - barbells, kettlebells, dumbbells and medicine balls are all great options.

Chapter Twenty-four

ONE THING

When I'm overwhelmed or truly have a lot on my plate, I like to step back and focus on one thing.

Basically, when everything is going a million miles per hour around you, it's pretty easy to look up at the end of the day and see that you're no closer to being happier or healthier than you were when the day started.

So rather than try to do a bunch of different things to improve, focus on ONE thing that will move you closer to your goals.

Now I'm not talking about the daily responsibilities of going to work, paying bills and taking care of your kids. Those are things that must be done.

But beyond that, make sure that you do ONE thing that makes you better and happier. It should also move you closer to your goals.

What do I mean?

- Be more engaged at meal time with how you are eating and who you are eating with.
- Apply something new that you have learned.
- Drink more water.

- Create a sleep ritual and stick to it.
- Move meaningfully and with a purpose for 20 minutes or more.
- Make each meal a little better... swap out potatoes for an extra serving of veggies, for example.

Even if the improvement is small, the power of this approach is big.

There is a compounding effect. Small successes build confidence, shape habits, and set you up for bigger wins down the road.

So, if you ever get overwhelmed with all there is to do (I know I do), then this is where I would start.

Focus on ONE thing at a time.

Chapter Twenty-five

FOCUS ON DONE

Y ou don't get results from a single workout or a couple of good meals. I've been lifting weights and exercising for a long time. I would rate workouts on a weekly basis as follows...

One will feel great.

A couple will be average to good.

And one will simply just go down in the books as 'done'.

I've learned that 'done' is what's most important. The combination of great, good, average, and bad is what leads to results. The sluggish workout days help maintain the compound gains you've been accruing from the average, good, and great days.

Even though that one workout may have sucked, you still showed up. You didn't chalk up a zero or skipped workout.

By simply showing up, you've proven that you aren't a person who misses workouts. Showing up has a powerful effect on your mindset, even when the workouts aren't that great.

A positive mindset keeps you coming back.

Decide to give your body some physical TLC and become a person who commits to it because you do what you say you are going to do.

Chapter Twenty-six

SWINGING FOR THE FENCES

Tomorrow is opening day for Major League Baseball. I watch little baseball, but opening day always reminds me of my baseball glory days.

Circa early 90s, I was a good high school baseball player. I was the starting varsity center fielder and leadoff batter all four years at Ely High. We were terrible my freshman year, but came one game away from state finals my junior year.

My job as a leadoff batter was to get on base. I was fast, had a good eye for balls and strikes, made good contact with the ball, and rarely struck out. In the baseball world, I was known as a "Punch and Judy." A slap hitter. A person who hits a lot of singles and doubles, but few home runs. I actually only hit two home runs my entire life during an official game. One during a Little League All-Star game (game-winning home run, thank you very much) and one against a neighboring rival in high school. You remember these things when there are so few.

Become a fitness Punch n' Judy.

We all love the home run. In fitness, the home run would be a new personal record in a lift, your fastest time in a run, or dropping a dress size.

Home runs are great, but long-term fitness is mostly about hitting singles. When you are putting good wood on the ball, hitting singles, the home runs will come. Good wood refers to making solid contact on the ball with the sweet part of the bat.

- Getting to the gym 3-4 times a week is hitting a single.
- Drinking a recovery protein shake after your training session is a single.
- Eating until you're 80% full is a single.
- If you are a runner, you have to log the miles. Just because a half marathon is 13.1 miles doesn't mean you always run that distance. A single would be getting out and crushing those 3 mile runs, paying attention to your gait and journaling what pre-run meal provided sustainable energy.
- Eating an adequate amount of protein each day is hitting a single.
- Working on a weakness is a single.
- Eating three servings of colorful vegetables each day is a single.
- Low to moderate intensity walks, bike rides or rowing sessions are singles.
- Meal planning and shopping are singles.
- Getting a good night's sleep is a single.

Your fitness home run is your ultimate reward. Your home run is a byproduct of consistent quality work and repetition. Day in and day out, you have to hit the singles. Focus on the little things and the big things will happen.

Make a list of "singles" that you need to hit daily to get you closer to your goal. Also, make a list of things that you need to avoid to keep you from slipping further away from your goal. We can only move in two directions. We always want to be taking more steps forward than backwards.

The first step is getting off the pine because nothing happens when you are sitting on the bench.

In baseball, riding the pine, means sitting on the bench.

Chapter Twenty-seven

JUST WIN BABY

I f you have a tendency to focus on the negative, you're not alone.

Sometimes, I fall into this trap, too.

I realized this while interviewing a prospective client recently. I asked, "What are you struggling with?"

This kind of language assumes that the person is struggling... it's a pretty negative place to begin a conversation, don't you think?

So, do your best not to start these negative conversations with yourself.

Focus on the positives.

Celebrate the wins, no matter how small.

A long-term accomplishment would be to say, "I lost 30 pounds!" That's certainly an achievement worth celebrating, but it will not happen today.

An achievement so impressive can't happen overnight, and there are no gimmicks or shortcuts that will get you there.

An achievement like that is really made up of a lot of small wins along the way. Things that might seem insignificant at the time, but that really add up in the long run.

So, my advice today is not to focus on the destination. Sure, dream big when you're setting your goals, but think small when it comes time to execute the little things each day that will lead to that achievement.

Did you meal prep last weekend? That's a win. Celebrate it.

Did you squeeze in a 15-minute home workout after you got stuck late at work? Another win. Give yourself a high-five.

Did you replace a second helping of rice with broccoli at dinner? Another seemingly small decision that, over time, will add up to big results.

Did you get seven hours of sleep last night? Do that consistently, and your body will thank you later. Both in ways that you can see (more muscle tone, less fat, healthier skin) and ways that you can't (healthier cells and hormonal balance).

So, along those lines, what's ONE SMALL WIN that you've had over the past week? It might be something that you didn't notice because you didn't think it mattered.

But now you know, it does.

A lot.

Chapter Twenty-eight

I THINK COACH IS TRYING TO KILL US

"Dom must have had a bad weekend" and "I think Coach is trying to kill us" are just a few phrases I sometimes overhear while walking through the gym during training sessions. For the record, I never let my personal life dictate a training program. And death would just be plain bad for business.

But I am a coach, and I love being a coach, which comes with responsibilities. Here are a few of my duties as a coach:

- Provide the path (the plan and a place to execute the plan).
- As Coach Dan John says, "Sometimes I get to sit back and be inspired by your effort and success. Other times I 'carry' you from here to there."
- Make fitness enjoyable by creating an environment that is comfortable and fun for our clients.
- Help clients come up with solutions that will help them reach their goals and improve their fitness and health.

Training programs that produce results

This is the duty that gets me dirty looks and leads to the above phrases. As a coach, it is my duty to find out how much you can handle. My team and I get a few days a week to help our clients improve their strength, conditioning and overall fitness. This means the sessions will be hard. You will be out of your comfort zone on the fringe. The fringe is where results are earned.

Each day, we try to recruit as much muscle fiber as possible. The more muscle fibers recruited, the better the result.

We will do this by working the entire body in each session. This recruitment of muscle will make your cardio-respiratory system respond. Your heart will pump blood at a rapid rate, and it will force your lungs to create oxygen. Your energy stores will get depleted. You'll be challenged appropriately, so that you can still function and be successful. Your body will feel fatigue and your muscles may get sore occasionally. Soreness is not the objective, but it sometimes comes with the territory.

It's science, but it ain't rocket science

There are training principles that need to be followed. Specificity, overload and progression matter. Within the boundaries of these laws, my options are limitless. If designed correctly, everything can work for a little while.

Factors that your coach should take into consideration

- What is your current fitness level? This tells me how much work you can handle.

- Do you have previous or current injuries? This tells me we need to be careful about how we program the work to be done.
- What is your biological age? A 70-year-old body handles stress differently than a 30-year-old body does.
- What is your training age? How long have you been lifting weights, running, and exercising? My training age is 30. I've been sprinting, jumping, running and lifting weights for 30 years. I will adapt and respond differently to someone new to the game. **New is an awesome time in the fitness game!**
- How is your sleep, nutrition, and water intake? These three items allow you to recover from the stress. If they stink, your training sessions may stink as well.
- How do you handle life stress? Work, family and our day-to-day... Is it under control?

Exercise is simply physical stress. A good stress. The body handles the stress or succumbs to it. When it handles the stress, it becomes stronger, leaner, and more resilient. This is the way.

The objective is to feel good from your sessions, see improvement, and enjoy the process. Great job to you, your coach, workout buddy or team if this is happening. But, if you feel miserable after your sessions and they are affecting other areas of life, then you need to consider finding another path.

Chapter Twenty-nine

GRANDPA'S COUGH SYRUP

"Coach, I want to drop 30lbs in three months, but I'm not giving up my wine."

"No problem, Lou Ann (fictional character). We have many members who enjoy wine and get excellent results. How much wine do you drink?"

"A bottle a night and more on the weekends. I've heard that a little wine each night has health benefits."

"Yes indeed. A little red wine may have health benefits. Broccoli has many health benefits as well. How much broccoli do you eat?"

"Oh, I don't like vegetables."

"I see."

If you've been reading my stuff, then you know I am not the coach who is constantly beating you over the head with Don'ts.

Like don't eat this or don't drink that. I prefer to help our members lay out a realistic plan that fits their lifestyle. For most, giving up alcohol or occasional treats is unrealistic.

Everything in moderation, right?

Indeed!

But, I've learned, everyone defines "moderation" a bit differently.

I enjoy drinking, and I know it can be part of a healthy lifestyle. I have witnessed members losing 20+lbs without giving up their booze completely. My intent of this article is to provide you with information on alcohol and how it may affect your fitness progress.

Here is what happens to your metabolism when you "skin back a few."

- You stop burning fat at a cellular level. The body doesn't store alcohol. When alcohol is ingested, it becomes the first priority for your metabolism. Your body will convert the alcohol into energy instead of using carbs and fats. So while you are drinking and shoveling in chicken nachos, it's a safe bet those nachos turn into back fat instead of useful energy.
- Your blood sugar takes a dip. Hooch temporarily "paralyzes" your liver's ability to make its own sugar, which causes a drop in blood sugar. Low blood sugar makes you crave simple carbs like Krispy Kreme donuts. Oh look! The hot light is on!
- Your growth hormone drops - alcohol causes this directly. Alcohol also affects sleep, which affects growth hormones as well.
- Your testosterone plummets - Alcohol increases the conversion of testosterone to estrogen in body fat- a process called aromatization.

- Excessive calories - A bottle of wine is roughly 25 ounces and 600+ calories. If you enjoy good beer, that's two beers - insert hysterically crying emoji.

I know what you are thinking. I can just add a couple of extra workouts in a week to burn the calories.

Forget about the calories!

The effect alcohol has on hormones, blood sugar and sleep is far more crucial.

If you are serious about losing fat and improving health, you may need to take a good look at your consumption of grandpa's cough syrup.

Chapter Thirty

NOT ENOUGH TIME

One of the most common complaints I hear from people who are struggling to stay on track with their fitness goals is, "I don't have time."

We all have time... it's just a matter of how we spend it.

This goes back to two factors:

1) Time Management; and

2) Mindset.

Let's start with mindset.

We are the only thing holding us back. I can talk myself in and out of anything. This holds true for most limiting beliefs. It's pretty damn easy to justify not doing something we don't want to do. And when we pursue something half-assed, it's also easy to make excuses for why we didn't succeed.

If you tell yourself at the outset that you don't have enough time to exercise and eat better, then you've already established a limiting belief that will guide your actions (or inaction).

A better approach would be to reprogram your brain with a new decision. It's always best to start small: "I believe that I have enough time to exercise 3 x per week. I can also pack leftovers as my lunch instead of ordering takeout with my co-workers."

The second aspect is how we view time. If we never seem to have enough time to do the things we "have to do," then maybe we should do fewer things.

It's also how we view the time that's required for exercise. At Breakthrough Fitness, we block out an hour for a client to complete their semi-private training session. If the client can't commit for an hour, we can accommodate and create 30-minute sessions. Workouts DO NOT need to be a specific length of time.

There will be days you get home late from work and can't make it to the gym or do a full-blown home workout. Instead of nothing, you could do a 10-minute training session of goblet squats and dumbbell presses, tracking how many sets you can get in during the 10 minutes.

Something I've done pretty well lately is meal-prep while the kids are taking showers. This gives me roughly 20-30 minutes in the evening to prepare for tomorrow night's dinner. Yes, I want to sit my ass down on the couch and chill, but I made a commitment to eating healthy. So, when I get the opportunity to break meal-prep into smaller, more manageable tasks, I do it.

Periods of ups and downs in your fitness are normal. What we don't want is off and on.

What are some minor changes you can make to time management?

With a little effort, do you think you can change your thoughts on exercise and eating well?

Focus on 1% better.

ON AND OFF

Circa 2005, I needed to get out of bartending. I was in and out of the fitness industry over the past five years. I did a little stint at a World's Gym, had an opportunity at a country club that could have been a good personal training gig, but I wasn't willing at the time to "put in the time." No doubt the easy cash- money I was making bartending had something to do with that.

My need to move on and be challenged led to my buddy Mike, who was in residential mortgages, introduced me to Diane, a realtor who was slinging houses big time in the area (I'm living in Pompano Beach at this time). In a few months, I went through the exam, paid the fees, and became a licensed realtor. I have a powerful memory of a lot of fees.

During this time, the real estate market was booming. Diane gave me a couple of handout deals. I helped a couple of friends buy houses and I was making progress and money. I can remember asking Diane what I should do? She would say in her high New York pitch, "What do you mean, just go get business!"

I could have used a little more direction, but now that I run my own business, Diane's voice is always in my head saying, "just go get business!" From Diane, I learned the importance of hustle and if you want to stay in business, new business is important.

Fast forward a few months and Diane opens a discount brokerage real estate office. This is great. I'm one of three agents on the ground floor. The downside was it was in Lake Worth, aka Lake Worthless.

I decided to go all in. No more bartending and I bought a townhouse in Lake Worth. The townhouse I bought a few years earlier has increased in value so much, I hopped on the real estate boom roller coaster.

The problem was that it all felt forced. I didn't like where I lived. I didn't like the relationship I was in. I didn't like my job.

And I didn't know it then, but I became depressed. I was the heaviest I've been, and I realized I haven't lifted weights and exercised in a year.

I knew I needed to get back to lifting and moving if I wanted to get out of this funk. I had to get back to the one constant that was in my life for the past fourteen years - lifting weights. Soon I was feeling better mentally, physically, and I was confident enough to make some tough decisions.

The girl went, and the house went up for sale (I was fortunate it sold because the winds of the real estate crash were at my door) and I was finished with selling real estate.

I was nervous and anxious, but my thoughts were positive. I felt good physically, and I had confidence and the willingness to "put in the time."

I made a commitment that my fitness would never be OFF again. It will always be On, with the flexibility to go Up and Down as needed.

You're on a ride through life, so you might as well do things that improve the ride. Strength training and heart-pumping exercise are great passengers. Start with untying them, taking the duct tape off their mouths and removing them from the trunk of the car.

Give them a chance.

Let them ride in the backseat and get to know them. Once comfortable, let them backseat occasionally. When it feels right, let them ride shotgun. You'll move them from the front seat to the back seat often. This is normal. The important part is not where they are sitting, but to enjoy their companionship on the ride.

Chapter Thirty-one

COFFEE AND...

My parents came to visit last week. After dinner the first evening my dad said to me, "We need to go to the store and buy some and." Confused, I asked, "What is and?" He said, "You know, coffee and.....a pastry, muffin or any kind of treat." Being cut from the same cloth as my father, I thought this was pretty funny. Over the next four days, our choice of nightly "And" became an important decision during the day.

You and "And"

And intake is completely individual. If your weight and physique are making you unhappy and you are working on improving your diet and fitness, then your consumption of And needs to be low.

Read that again.

I said low. You are allowed to eat And. I've seen no one be successful at changing their physique without enjoying themselves a little, and once in a while.

Life is too short not to be happy. If weight gain, lack of energy and being out of shape have you feeling blue, do what is necessary to find your happy place. Don't forget to enjoy the journey, for that is where you will find happiness.

Maintaining a healthy weight while enjoying And

Everyone is unique and your lifestyle will dictate how much And you can consume without gaining weight. Remember that And can affect more than just weight. Health factors like blood pressure and cholesterol can be negatively impacted by And.

My dad loves some And. Let's see how he has been able to manage his weight and health in his 70s.

- Every morning my dad and stepmom take the dogs for a brisk 2-3 mile walk.
- He maintains his house- landscaping in the summer, snow plowing in the winter (he lives in Connecticut).
- Every evening, those beloved dogs get another 2-3 mile walk. Unless they are snowed in or the temperatures are extremely low, these walks take place. *Note to all my Floridians - A temperature of 60 degrees is not considered extremely low.
- Three meals are eaten daily and 99.5% of the time they are prepared at home. My parents watch their salt intake. They do not eat a lot of packaged rice or other processed foods.
- Meals usually comprise meat, starch, vegetables, and does not drink sodas or alcohol.
- And is NOT consumed every night.
- When And is eaten, it is a small piece.

- Observing and taking part in my dad's And intake would lead me to the conclusion that 10% of his daily calories are coming from And.

Plan the And

How you enjoy And is up to you. If you are someone who enjoys adult beverages and frequents restaurants regularly, additional And over a time will lead to weight gain.

If you live a lifestyle like my dad and tossed in 3-4 intense strength training sessions a week, your physique should be quite nice. The best way to change your physique and allow for a little And is to plan for it.

I like the 80/20 rule for a healthy lifestyle.

80% of the time you are eating foods that are found in nature, close to their original form - veggies, fruits, animal protein sources, whole grains, nuts and seeds.

20% of the time - the other stuff.

Let's say you can eat 2000 calories a day to maintain your current weight.

20% = 400 calories (2000 x 20%)

That's a lot of calories for the "other stuff".

Now, if you are trying to lose fat, you may want to drop the And down to 10-15%

That still allows 200-300 calories for coffee And...

Chapter Thirty-two

THE ULTIMATE EDGE IN FAT LOSS

During his first meeting with a new team, legendary basketball coach John Wooden would have all the players take off their socks and shoes. He would then make the team put their socks back on meticulously, making sure that every wrinkle was out of the sock. He knew basketball was a game of quick movement and direction change. This was hard on the feet. A wrinkled sock can cause blisters. Blisters can lead to loss of playing time, which could hurt the team's winning chances.

Details matter.

Fiber is the wrinkled sock in the game of fat loss. It's a minor detail that can have a big impact on your chance of winning.

Fiber itself does not burn fat, but it can help tremendously in our efforts to lose fat.

What is fiber?

- Fiber is nothing more than a carbohydrate that the body can not digest.
- There are two types: Insoluble fiber and soluble fiber.

Insoluble Fiber

- Does not dissolve in water.
- Helps move food through the digestive system.
- Promotes regularity and helps prevent constipation.

Soluble Fiber

- Dissolves in water.
- Soluble fiber lowers blood sugar levels and lowers cholesterol levels.

How can fiber help with fat loss⬚?

- High-fiber foods do not contain as much digestible carbohydrate, so it slows the rate of digestion and causes a more gradual and lower rise in blood sugar.
- Slower digestion keeps you full longer.
- The 'Chew Factor' - High fibrous foods take longer to eat. This gives the brain enough time to get the signal that you are full.

Strive for 25

Try to eat 25-30 grams per day.

Foods high in fiber

- Raspberries - 8g per cup
- Blackberries - 7g per cup
- Avocado - 6g per 1/2
- Pears - 5g medium fruit
- Peas - 8g per cup
- Broccoli - 5g per cup
- Sweet potato w/skin - 6g medium potato
- Black beans - 8g 1/2 cup
- Lentils - 8g 1/2 cup

- Oatmeal - 4g per cup
- Quinoa - 5g per cup
- Brown rice - 4g per cup

Notice what all these foods have in common? They are all carbohydrates!

Do you think you would lose fat if:

- Your diet comprised the above foods, paired with good protein and fats.
- You controlled portions, so your daily calories match the amount of calories you need per day.
- You lifted weights and did circuit training a few days a week.
- You did low intensity movement a couple of days a week.
- You eased off the wine, beer and alcohol.
- You backed off the dairy.
- You took a "get better" not "perfect" approach to eating.

Hell yes you would!

Look at Strive for 25 as the next big thing, the new shiny object.

Because if you eat 25+ grams of fiber every day, you'll see and feel the results.

Important Tips

Fiber absorbs water, so you want to make sure you are drinking adequate amounts of water when you increase fiber intake.

- Try to get most of your fiber from fruits, vegetables and legumes.
- The rest should come from whole grains - oatmeal, rice, quinoa.
- Beware of foods disguised as healthy. DO NOT rely on packaged food sources for your fiber. Most of it is junk food masquerading around as if it's good for you.

Chapter Thirty-three

FREE WEIGHTS OR MACHINES?

Over the last 27 years, I have used an array of barbells and dumbbells, numerous leg machines, a host of pulley machines, and a diverse selection of weight-plate loaded machines. I've used medicine balls, kettlebells, suspension straps (TRX, gymnastic rings), stability balls, resistance bands, sleds and ropes.

As you can see, there is no shortage of equipment out there to use. So which is better: the free weights or machines?

It depends.

You can build strength, endurance, and change the shape of your muscles using both free weights and machines. But which one is right for you depends on a few different factors.

- Goals
- Access
- Enjoyment

Law of Specificity: you get what you train

A professional bodybuilder's goal is to have the biggest, well-balanced, ripped physique. This type of training requires lots of volume and muscular fatigue. Machines can be a good choice, since form may break down when we push to failure and beyond.

A grandma who wants to lift, carry and move around freely with her grandchildren would probably benefit more from free weights since we can replicate the movements she wants to do: squat, bend, carry, and lift.

Access

If you already have a few sets of dumbbells that you've been using forever, there's no reason to buy a fancy machine. If your gym has only machines (or if the free weights are always in use), do the machines.

The best workout is one you'll actually do. You'll get results by showing up and doing the necessary work.

Enjoyment

What kind of movement and strength training do you enjoy the most?

As I said earlier, the best workout is the one you actually do. If you hate lifting free weights, don't force yourself to use them. If you dislike the fixed movement of a machine, step away and use dumbbells and TRX straps.

Free weights most of the time

I don't think anyone can really argue that our society needs more free, natural movement daily.

When more movement is part of the equation, I feel it should be done with free weights. I also think the first weight we should learn to use is our body - **the ultimate free weight!**

I like the learning curve that comes with free weights. You are forced to pay attention to the movement. Over time, your body adapts and coordinates the multiple actions that need to take place for smooth movement.

There is a hidden benefit to grabbing a pair of dumbbells off of the rack, laying back on a bench, hoisting them up to the start position, performing the prescribed repetitions and safely getting the weights to the floor. Then, when it's time to repeat, bend over, grip the weights firmly, create tension through the body, and hoist them back up.

There is a lot of value in getting down on the floor for planks, bird dogs, hip bridges and crawling exercises.

Carries- walking for distance or time with a heavy weight in your hand(s) builds grip strength like nothing else. A strong grip is a sign of vitality and vigor.

There are research studies that conclude grip strength is a predictor of muscular endurance and overall strength. Also, studies have found that a stronger grip correlates with a lower risk of heart attack and stroke.

Machines are tools in your tool box

Just because it's a good exercise doesn't mean it's good for you. Pull-ups are fantastic for building upper body strength, but are they for you? Do you have shoulder problems? Are you just getting into fitness? Are you a middle-aged person like me?

I have a threshold on how many pull-ups I can do in a training session. When I go over my limit, my elbows hurt and a past collarbone injury flares up. So, while I can still do them, I prefer a variety of pull-downs and rowing patterns that can be done on machines. **An excellent program should never ask you to do something you can't do pain-free.**

Every aspect of fitness and life improves from strength. You could say, strength training is "everything" training, so have fun and use a variety of free weights and machines. The best thing you can do is experiment and try new things. The body enjoys moving in a variety of ways.

As you try new things, be sure to add them one at a time. See how it goes for a while, then decide about whether it's useful. If it is not useful, toss it aside and move on.

Chapter Thirty-four

THE SAUSAGE STAND

This Sunday, while my family and I made the rounds at the usual suspects- Home Depot, Pet Supermarket and Costco, I ran into someone I've met on many occasions. Our paths crossed at the exit of Home Depot where the savory smell of sausage creates Homer Simpson like reactions... Ummm sausage. The timing was classic. As she turned, eyes closed, mouth open wide, she passionately took the first bite. Her eyes soon opened, only to be flooded by guilt as our gaze met. A wave of guilt hit me as well because I never wanted to ruin the first bite of a delicious sausage!

Her guilt wasn't because I frowned at eating sausage. I'm like Abe Froman when it comes to sausage (Ferris Bueller's Day Off reference for those lost on this one). Her guilt lied in the fact that all of our past conversations had to do with her asking me for advice on losing weight, which I am always happy to oblige. She knew this wasn't an "I'm going to enjoy a sausage because I've eaten really well all week" moment.

This was, "I haven't eaten breakfast and now I'm starving, let me grab the first thing convenient" moment.

Though it could have been an "I just can't resist eating sausage every time I smell sausage" moment. I'm not completely sure. I never set out to be the guy to ruin someone's moment of indulgence. Then I started to think, maybe it's a good thing I can cause a feeling of guilt. We're grown adults- you know you don't need a sausage every time you encounter one. Especially if you're trying to lose weight. If I can, for only a few seconds hold you accountable, fantastic.

Accountability is a key to success. I have a business coach. Why? Because it's easy to do stuff, that's meaningless and sabotaging. My coach knows my goals, knows what I need to do to obtain those goals, and helps me stay focused on meaningful activities.

If you are looking to improve your fitness and health, it starts by building an accountability team and creating the right environment that nurtures improvement.

Invest in yourself by hiring a fitness coach or a facility that surrounds you with people just like you. Ask your fit friend for advice- they'll be happy to help. Join a running club with a friend or just show up and make new friends. Stop trying to do it alone.

And If you can't resist sausage, leave through the gardening exit and make a mad dash to your vehicle, never looking back until you're safely out of the parking lot.

Chapter Thirty-five

STOP THE HATE

Y ou can't hate yourself healthy.

I've talked before about the three things that need to change if you want to see improvements in your body, health and overall happiness.

1. Think right - mind, attitude, mood.
2. Eat right - lots of veggies and protein is a great place to start.
3. Move right - strength training lays the foundation. They might seem like separate entities, but they're all intertwined. Movement and highly nutritious foods have a positive effect on our mood and mindset. But they can't erase the demons or mental struggles you are dealing with from your childhood, past relationships, and your own perceptions.

I've witnessed clients eat right, move right and think right for periods of time, only to let doubt, lack of confidence and hateful talk about their bodies and character crush their chance for results to stick.

Negative self-talk will become a self-fulfilling prophecy.

Pay close attention to how you talk to yourself and others about - your body, food, and working out.

Your actions and your speaking have to match. It's time to *flip the script*....

You could say, *"I can never resist when you guys bring baked goods to work."*

Or

"You guys are going to have to eat the brownies without me this time. I don't eat brownies on Tuesday lol. Don't worry, I'll make sure to have something sweet on my free day."

The ride to improvement starts with movement.

Lift weights, sweat and breath heavily sometimes.

Get outside and play with the kids/grandkids, go for casual walks and take the boat out more often.

Eat more vegetables, get more pedicures, and laugh daily.

Start moving and let the magical powers seep into your brain, creating thoughts of strength, confidence, and vigor.

Keep moving forward, embracing and confronting things head on.

There's beauty in the struggle.

Chapter Thirty-six

CLOSING

Congratulations, you've reached the end of the book. I want to believe that you read every word, had a few aha moments and even a few laughs. But, I know it's possible you read the first page, skimmed a few stories and are now here reading these last words.

Either way, I'm happy the book is in your hands.

Now, I want to help you turn the lessons from this book and the knowledge you already have into action.

Fitness and improving eating habits can be challenging because life is going to happen.

Unfortunately, life doesn't stop happening just because you decide to start a workout plan or eat a few more vegetables.

That's why coaching and community are so important. A coach and members of your fitness community will hold you accountable, keeping you moving forward.

And it's way more fun!

So, here's a gift to get you started!

Finding a coach or team of coaches and the right facility is something you shouldn't take lightly. That's why we want you to come in and experience Breakthrough Fitness. We want you to get a feel for our environment, work through your programs and interact with the coaches and other members to see if it's the right fit for you.

Call now to activate your gift card and to set up your Breakthrough Strategy Session.

407-542-5910

Keep moving,

Coach Dom

ABOUT THE AUTHOR

Dominic Lucibello is a nutrition and fitness coach who specializes in helping people cut through the confusion of fitness and fat loss.

He is the founder of Breakthrough Fitness in Oviedo, Florida, where for the past 12 years his team has helped hundreds of clients upgrade their lives through better nutrition and consistent strength training. His weekly fitness articles and stories are read by thousands of regular readers. When he's not coaching, he's spending time with his wife and two children. Please visit his website at - www.breakthroughfitnessfl.com

Made in the USA
Columbia, SC
31 October 2023